Back Pain Relief and the Spinal Cord Stimulator Implant

How I went from a back injury to relief with a SCS implant

By
Russ Lawson, PhD.
10/02/2018

Dedication

To **Dr. Craig Critchley** who started me on this journey
and cared for me in the beginning.
To **Dr. Lance Tigyer** who advised me and did the surgery
and implanted the stimulator.
To **Laura Harlow** who advises; programs and maintains
my stimulator implant.
To **Judy Crow** who read through the proof copy and made
some good suggestions.

But most especially:
To the love of my life for these past 51 years, my wife
Melody who has shown a special kind of patience and
kindness and who has learned to nurse me and care for me
even when I'm grumpy.

ISBN: 9781728880976

Introductory Thoughts:

I am not a medical doctor, although I do hold 2 PhD's. What that basically says about me is that I am a researcher. When I become involved in something I dig into it and find out everything I can and weigh my options before making a decision. That's what I did with my decision to receive a Spinal Cord Simulator implant.

Why this book?

Why take the time to write this book? Because when I started my journey to learn about Spinal Cord Stimulators (SCS), I could find very little written about them. Most of what you could read was on the manufactures websites and I read those with some doubt as they obviously want to promote their product.

What you will read here is my journey. I will try and help you understand my physical condition, what I learned through my research and how things have worked out for me, perhaps they will work for you, but ultimately it is your decision. I went from pain and walking with a cane to a pretty much normal life. I encourage you to become a researcher also, study your options, interview people who have had this treatment and make your own decision. I give you the tools to do this here in this book.

I will define what I can and give a few links to websites, blogs and/or forums that you might find helpful. But most of all I will be honest with you and try to answer some of the questions I had regarding SCS. I had a lot of questions and it took a lot of digging before I was satisfied that this was the right decision. I did my own research, interviewed people who had the implant procedure and then drew my own conclusions. I hope this will help you as you try and do the same.

Disclaimer:

I have to be up front with you and let you know that ***Federal Regulations prohibits me*** from claiming that I have medical training or from offering medical advice. I am only sharing my experiences and research in this area.

Also, understand that I strongly recommend that you spend time with your health care professional before using any product that claims to be of health benefit.

You can choose to ignore this advice, but you do so at your own risk. My only purpose is to share what has benefited me and others. Also, understand that each and every one of us is different; our bodies don't react the same all of the time, what works for me, may not work as well for you. So, proceed with whatever you choose to do with caution. Do your research, check with professionals because after all you literally do hold your life in your own hands.

A little bit about me… background

In 2015 I, (semi), retired from being a full time minister and former missionary to Africa. After around 48 years in full time ministry in different areas of the world, (from New Hampshire to California), my wife and I decided it was time to come back to our birthplace in Ohio. Our families, children and especially our grandchildren were there and we wanted to be involved in their lives before they out grew us.

I had managed to earn two PhD's, (ministry and education) and become a Certified Family Herbalist also. So, as I said before, I am a researcher and a lifelong learner also. Besides that I am a writer. I have written a column for a small town newspaper for 16 years and a blog for about as along. I also have written 7 books and numerous study guides for distance learning. Some you can find on Amazon.com and some on lulu.com.

My Journey begins…..

After my semi-retirement I have continued to preach occasionally, but also took a secular job which for the most part I enjoyed and found to be challenging. It was somewhat physically demanding, but I never shied away from physical work.

In 2016 I began to have back problems, however I didn't realize it was my back that was the seat of my problems. It began with an attack of Sciatica in my left leg. Pain, weakness, limping, more pain, numbness…. I made an appointment with my family doctor who gave me a steroid injection and pain relievers. I saw him again after a week and he sent me for physical therapy at a Sports Medicine Rehab center. I went there 2 times a week for about 4 months. I had massage, heat, electrical stimulation and physical exercise and eventually regained the use of my leg, mostly pain free.

At the time I was working for a major home improvement store which was physically demanding at times and always called for a lot of physical activity. On a normal day I would walk from 3 to 7 miles in the store. I moved lumber, filled orders, hauled washers, dryers, refrigerators, pulled material for building contractors as well as worked behind the desk and cash register.

At home I cut my own grass, did my own yard work and all of our household repairs. Now, all of that is to say again that I had a very physically demanding lifestyle. I might add that I am 70 years old and in fairly good shape though a little over weight. I take no meds at all other than herbs and supplements. A doctor's visit was a rare thing and some years only going for a yearly checkup.

Having said that, you can imagine how disturbing it was to be cut off from physical activity, but perhaps you are there yourself.

In 2017 I began to have more problems, this time it was my right leg. I awoke on the morning of September 16th with excruciating pain in my lower back and right leg. So much so, that my wife had to drive me to the emergency room for and exam and treatment. I had been moving boxes of ceiling fans at my job the day before and feel that was as they say, "the straw that broke the camels back". At the Emergency room they checked me out and thought it was my sciatic nerve again though on the other side of my body. They gave me some high powered pain meds and told me to follow up with me family doctor, which I did.

My family doctor is an excellent doctor and did a through physical evaluation and once again gave me a steroid injection and sent me for x-rays. His diagnosis was also that it was a sciatic nerve problem. At my follow up appointment he said the x-rays showed that I had 3 bulging disks and below them 3 compressed disks in my lower back with a mild Spinal Stenosis (narrowing of the spinal cord channel).

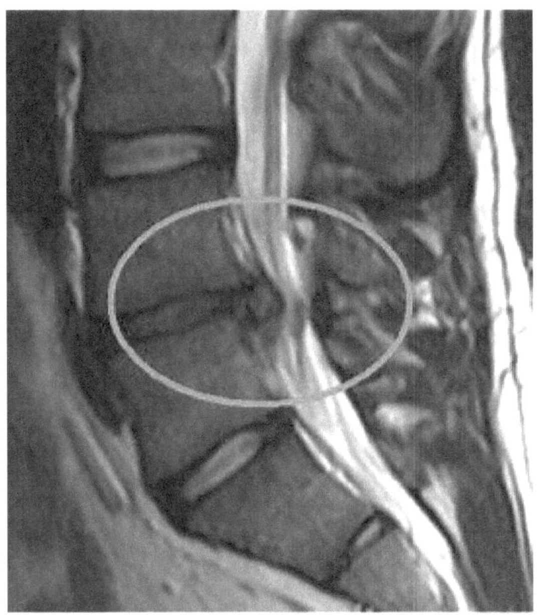
Bulging disk

Next he wanted to send me for an MRI, but the way he explained it to me was, since I am insured by Medicare they will not allow that until after 6 weeks of treatment. So, he sent me back to physical therapy again. This time the pain just did not go away. I did get some relief, but was walking with a cane because my right leg would give out on me unexpectedly and fell a few times. I also had numbness and tingling in my toes.

I might add that from this point I was unable to return to work. I was only able to stand for 15 to 20 minutes and with the pain and weakness in my leg I was reduced to laying in bed most of the time for several weeks other than going to my physical therapy and doctor appointments.

The physical therapy was a little more aggressive this time and they also administered something called "Dry Needling." Dry Needling is much like Acupuncture, but designed to stimulate blood flow in the area that had the nerve damage with the purpose of promoting healing. It gave a little temporary relief, but nothing lasting.

The therapist eventually tried stretching my spine in the hopes of relieving the pressure on the nerves. This involved tying off my upper body and hanging weights off of a contraption hooked to my hips, but rather than helping it gave me more pain. I had to refuse that treatment after that incident.

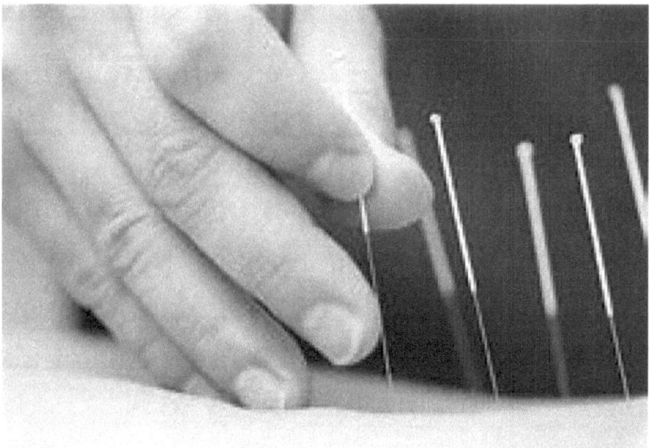

Dry Needling

The MRI

My family doctor was finally able to send me for an MRI (Magnetic Resonance Imaging).

Definition: *MRI*

A MRI is - a noninvasive diagnostic technique that produces computerized images of internal body tissues and is based on nuclear magnetic resonance of atoms within the body induced by the application of radio waves —called also MRI.

My Results:

The results were a little more specific which allowed me to seek further treatment. I don't claim to understand all of the wording, but depended upon my doctors to explain it all to me.

From the report: ***"Patient has weakness in the right hip with low back pain shooting down his leg to the knee. Right leg gives out, using a cane, some numbness in feet."***

"Conclusion: L1 – L5 – S1, Disk desiccation. Shallow central disk displacement L4-5 without central canal Stenosis or thecal sac compression. Mild central canal Stenosis L2-3 level with moderate foraminal narrowing effacing the exiting L2 nerve root in combination with facet arthropathy."

Definition: _Disk Desiccation_:

The definition of disc desiccation is a degenerative disc disease that occurs when the fluid between spinal discs dries out. When the protein-like substance that surrounds spinal discs is gone, the spine becomes unable to support the weight of a body, and flexibility and mobility are severely...

Definition: _Facet arthropathy_:
Your body's facet joints are the joints on the back of your spine that counterbalance the disks inside your spine's vertebrae. They're important for limiting the motion of your spine so that the vertebrae stay in proper alignment.

Over time, aging causes the facet joints to wear down. Arthritis of these joints may also occur over time, just as it might in any other joint. This is referred to as facet arthropathy
 People with facet arthropathy often experience lower back pain that worsens with twisting, standing, or bending backward. This pain is usually centered on one specific part of the spine. It may also feel like a dull ache on one or both sides of the lower back.

Unlike the pain of a slipped disk or sciatica, facet arthropathy pain typically doesn't radiate into your buttocks or down your legs. However, the joint can become enlarged, like any other joint that has arthritis, and press on nerve roots that could cause pain to radiate down your lower extremity.

Facet arthropathy pain is typically relieved by bending forward. The pressure, or load, on your facet joints is reduced when you bend your body forward into a spinal flexion position. (Note: this definition from www.Healthline.com).

The Specialist:

So, what does this all mean? Well according to my family doctor it means that I have some disk compression, some bulging disks, some narrowing of the spinal canal and a little arthritis in my spine.

Since I now had the MRI results my family doctor referred me to a specialist, (the same one who had worked on him). The specialist is an orthopedic surgeon who specializes in backs. So, an appointment was made and the next step in this journey began.

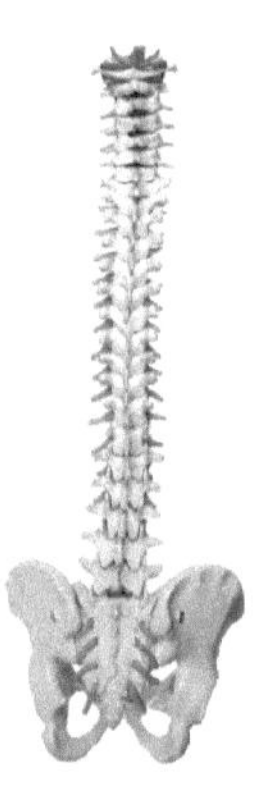

The orthopedic surgeon

I had been dealing with the pain and debilitation now for over two months, my short term disability from my employer was running out and I desperately wanted to get some answers and hopefully some relief from my pain. If you have been going through this you probably know I was overly optimistic that this would be a fairly quick fix. It just doesn't happen that way.

My appointment began with the usual questions by the nurse then a trip to their x-ray department. After that back to the exam room where the doctor eventually came in and this new leg of my journey began.

The doctor asked the normal questions and did a short physical exam, examined the MRI and x-rays, etc. When he finished he gave me the bad news. His comments were something like this:

"Mr. Lawson, with your type of injury there is really nothing I can do to fix things. I could suggest surgery, but it is my experience that in cases like this it does not help and sometimes makes things worse. At this point I can offer some treatments that may give you relieve from some of the pain, but pain management is about the best we can do."

I was both impressed and disappointed at the same time. I was impressed that a surgeon would tell me that surgery in my case would basically be a waste of time and disappointed that he couldn't make me "all better".

He then discussed some options with me for pain management. He talked about pain meds, epidural injections, and surgery to implant a Spinal Cord Stimulator.

I dismissed the idea of the Spinal Cord Simulator without really giving it any consideration. Through my years of being a minister and sometimes spending as much time in hospitals as do doctors, I had heard too many disappointing stories involving back surgeries.

Lumbar Epidural Steroid Injections

I did agree to try the epidural injections and scheduled one for the next available appointment. They are called: Lumbar Epidural Steroid Injections, and are given for Low Back Pain and Sciatica. Most of the time this is only a temporary fix, but I have spoken with some who have had permanent relief from this procedure.

What is an epidural steroid injection?

"An epidural steroid injection (ESI) is the delivery of powerful anti-inflammatory medicine directly into the space outside of the sac of fluid around your spinal cord. This area is called the epidural space." (www.medlineplus.com)

For the actual procedure they have you lay on your stomach. They then set up a fluoroscope to watch the procedure as they actually perform it.

Fluoroscope [floor′o-skōp″]
An instrument for visual observation of the body by means of X-RAY.
> The patient is put into position so that the part to be viewed is placed between an x-ray tube and a fluorescent screen. X-rays from the tube pass through the body and pr oject the bones and organs as images on the screen. Examination by this method is called fluoroscopy.

The advantage of the fluoroscope is that the action of joints, organs, and entire systems of the body can be observed directly.

The use of radiopaque media and radiolucent agents aids in this process.
https://medical-dictionary.thefreedictionary.com

This allows them to take the long thin needles and insert them between your disks and inject the medication accurately where needed. They do give you mild local before the procedure and for me this first procedure was only mildly uncomfortable.

Did it work?

Did it work for me? Yes and no. Yes it helped relieve the pain to some degree, but not all of the pain magically disappeared. It was more like portions of my back were numb on the outside, but he deep pain still remained. I remember trying to describe it to my wife. I said, "When taking a shower I can use warm water on my back, but my lower back where they injected me has no sensation on the skin, the water feels cold."

How did this affect me?

At this point the doctor had me on a limit of lifting no more than 10 pounds and he wanted me to gct a cane with the 3 or 4 feet on it for more stability. (I was limping badly and sometimes my leg gave out. I had fallen a couple of times.) But the doctor also encouraged me to walk when I could. And follow up with him. The injections really did not improve my quality of life at all. If they helped at all, it was only for a few days.

The doctor suggested that I take another round of injections as it sometimes took 2 or 3 treatments to see some substantial results. So, after about 4 weeks they preformed the procedure again, this time trying to be more specific in the areas they injected me. They questioned me more thoroughly about just where the pain was at and tried to center in to those areas as much as possible.

The results for me were just the same, maybe a little relief for a couple of days, but nothing substantial or lasting.

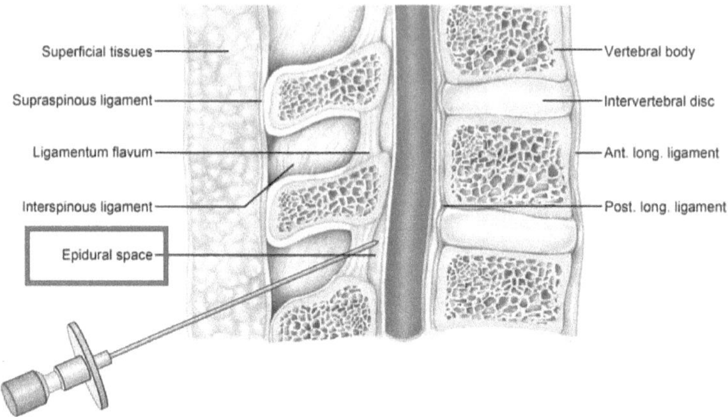

Epidural Injection

My next step…

I returned to my family doctor and explained my disappointment at my inability to find an answer or get any permanent relief. I ask him if he could recommend someone for a second opinion which he did.

The referral was to another doctor which also specialized in back pain. He once again sent me for x-rays and then had a consultation with him. He gave me the same diagnosis as the first doctor. There was nothing he could do for me, but referred me to a pain management clinic. So, I made that appointment and that led me to where I am today.

Pain Management Clinic

I have to say that I was super impressed with the doctor at the pain management clinic. He spent about 2 hours with me and gave me the most through physical exam of any of the doctors. There also were 14 pages of forms to fill out before the exam. You could see a theme as they asked several times if I used opiates, how often, etc. They also asked at least 4 times if I had ever considered suicide or was ever depressed. I had refused any opiates and was only taking Tylenol or Ibuprofen at the time and had never been depressed about the situation, so we didn't have a problem.

I might mention that at one point one of my doctors asked me if I was having any problem with depression and suggested that there were pills that could help if I were. I told him no, that wasn't necessary. For me that was never an issue, I have a great support network in my family and my church.

An Introduction to the world of Spinal Cord Stimulators

What is a Spinal Cord Stimulator?

It is a device that has been developed for people with chronic back pain. It is implanted in the lower back with wire leads inserted into the area around spinal cord canal. It uses electrical pulses to stimulate nerves in the spinal cord. Basically it interferes with the path of pain signals as they travel to the brain. In most cases you can adjust the level of stimulation and in some cases the areas that the stimulation effects.

Let me mention that the Spinal Cord Stimulator is **not for everyone**. There is of course your specific physical problem, but there is also the question of whether you can manage the daily operation of the unit. You have a personal remote that allows you to control programs in the unit and then you will need to charge the internal battery of the implant as well as the controls. Depending on how much you use the unit, the intensity settings, etc. will determine how often you will need to charge the units. Not everyone can handle these challenges in the daily operation.

Take a look at the implant:

You can find images on line, but I like how this one shows in detail what is going on with a stimulator placement.

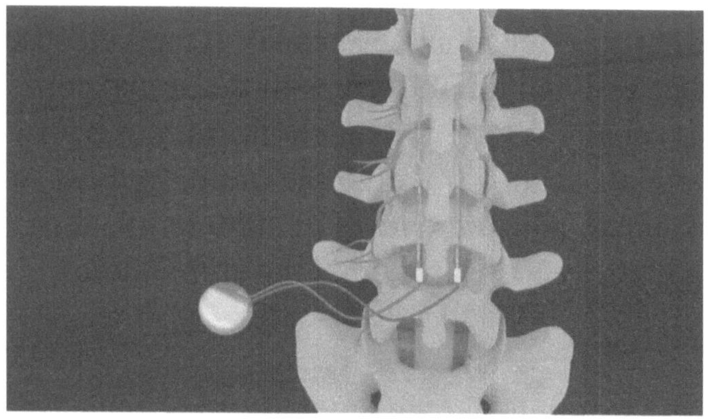

A better graphic can be seen at the links below.

Graphic from Website – Click here to go to:
http://www.bostonscientific.com/en-US/patients/health-conditions/chronic-pain.html

Graphic from Website – Click here or go to:
http://nuvectramedical.com/us/patient/about-scs/

Some of the things I learned

One of the things they did at the pain clinic was to
spend a little time talking to me about the option of
a Spinal Cord Stimulator Implant (SCS). They gave
me a packet with some information and a DVD in it,
but it really didn't give me the in-depth information
my research background demanded. What it did do
was give me a place to start.

I found out that there were a number of steps that
had to be taken before your insurance would
consider you for the Spinal Cord Stimulator and all
but one of them I had already accomplished.

1. There had to be a period of time pass where
    traditional treatment was tried.

2. You had to have tried the epidural injections.

3. Therapy was required by some.

4. An MRI, x-rays, as well as physical exams
    must be submitted to prove that there was
    truly an issue that could be aided by the
    implant.

5. You had to have a psychological evaluation
    to determine if you were mentally able to deal
    with the implant. Part of the evaluation I had
    dealt with whether or not I was dealing with
    dementia. (The Spinal Cord Stimulator has a

remote control which you as the patient need to monitor and control as your personal needs and activities dictate as well as charging the individual parts of the units).

6. You would have to have a temporary, (test), implant of leads into your spinal column with the sending unit/ computer taped to your side for 3 to 5 days. The purpose is to see whether or not the SCS would work for you.

A few days after my visit to the Pain Clinic a representative from Boston Scientific called me. They were very gracious and informative as they told me more about their device and answered some questions for me. I was very impressed at this personal contact. But then I was still exploring my options.

There is more than one choice

One of the first things I learned was that there are choices when it comes to Spinal Cord Stimulators. They have actually been doing this type of implant for the past 40 years and have literally done millions of these procedures.

There are several different major companies which manufacture Spinal Cord Stimulators. I really couldn't tell much difference between them and what they do when I began, but my research continued. Below is a basic introduction to a few of these companies.

- Boston Scientific (formerly known as Advanced Bionics) entered the market in 2004 with the first 16 contact system, each with an independent current source. This is one of the most used companies it seemed to me. They have a great reputation and those I spoke with who have this unit have been happy with it.

- Medtronic working with Avery Labs in 1972 commercialized the first spinal cord stimulator system.

- St. Jude Medical (formerly known as ANS – Advanced Neuromodulation Systems) in 1986 released the first 8 contact system under the corporate name of Neuromed.

Again, those who have this unit seem to be very happy with it also.

- <u>NuVectra/Algovita,</u> The Algovita® Spinal Cord Stimulation System combines the best aspects of proven Spinal Cord Stimulator technology (http://nuvectramedical.com/) into a single, patient-friendly system. It enables you to customize pain therapy to your individual needs, so you can get back to living the active life you want.

Comparison Chart

Boston Scientific put together a partial comparison chart that you can find here, but it does not contain the NuVectra information:

https://www.neuromodlearning.com/NLI/assets/File/NM-237708-AB_SCS%20System%20Comparison%20Chart_Final.pdf

NuVectra website here with more information about there unit: http://nuvectramedical.com/

Personal Notes on my choice:

Not all doctors' deal with all of the different equipment manufacturers. If you have a preference you will need to check with the manufacturer and see what doctors' in your area use their equipment. I actually called my doctors office and asked specifically what Stimulator they used.

Understand that you do not have to stay with one doctor or stimulator brand. It is your body and you have the right to make a choice in this matter. It may be that you feel that you are not qualified to make that decision and that is fine. That is why we have doctors, to help us by making educated recommendations for us.

The Pain Clinic where I went actually used the Boston Scientific unit. I researched this unit very deeply. I was very impressed and was all ready to go with this unit, but then I ran across the NuVectra/Algovita system. In my mind it offers just a little bit more, but I'm sure the Boston Scientific unit would have done very well for me also.

I did decide to go with a doctor that offered the **NuVectoa/Algovita** system. Surprisingly enough it was offered by the original Orthopedic Surgeon I had first seen.

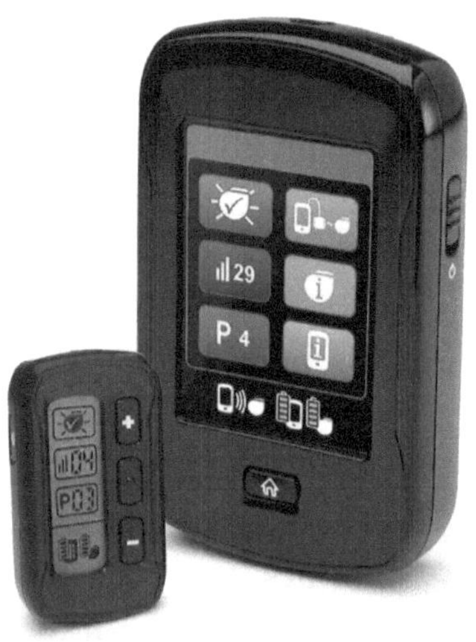

An example of some of the components for controlling and charging the implant

More Research

Following is a copy of one of the articles that helped sway me in this direction.

SANTA CLARA, Calif. — January 5, 2017 — Based on its recent analysis of the spinal cord stimulation (SCS) market, Frost & Sullivan recognizes Nuvectra with the 2017 North American New Product Innovation Award for its flagship product, the Algovita® SCS System. SCS is fast becoming the non-drug alternative for chronic pain conditions, and Nuvectra's commitment to advancing next-generation neurostimulation technologies makes it a crucial player in the market.

"The multi-billion-dollar global chronic pain management market is significantly underserved," explained Frost & Sullivan Global Director, Venkat Rajan. "Chronic pain affects over a 100 million people in the United States (US) and conventional treatments primarily rely on opioid use, which poses risks that include reduced function, addiction, overdose, and even death. On the other hand, neurostimulation therapies, and SCS in particular, have garnered a reputation as an effective and safe treatment for refractory chronic pain over the past four decades."

Nuvectra's Algovita® system uniquely combines electronic architecture, implantable pulse generator

(IPG) capabilities, and wireless telemetry to enable agile, individually tailored SCS therapy for a range of chronic pain patients. It allows physicians to design multiple treatment programs, empowering patients to select therapy options based on daily pain experiences. Moreover, Algovita®'s upgradable and expandable platform is designed to be responsive to market changes, potentially providing non-invasive updates to implement the latest therapies for optimal care.

"The SCS sector in the United States will be at nearly $1.5 billion by 2018 and although it is a mature market, increasing disease prevalence, demand for innovative therapies, and wider patient acceptance will drive high market growth," observed Rajan. "Nuvectra's broad-based neurostimulation platform positions the company for accelerated future growth. Its improved therapy delivery system, including enhanced features for a simple physician and patient user experience coupled with the platform's powerful, upgradable versatility, will enable different therapeutic approaches and markets."

Pain physicians or neurosurgeons conduct 3- to 7-day trials using percutaneous leads to evaluate the individual benefit for each patient. Once SCS is found to be a viable option for the patient, implantation of the IPG is done. Thereafter, physicians and Nuvectra representatives work to set the therapy configuration that effectively relieves patients of their pain. While physicians appreciate Algovita®'s breadth of capabilities, usability, and the ease of lead implantation, patients like the system's effectiveness and the portable programmer's easy-to-use interface.

CE marked and approved by the Food and Drug Administration (FDA), Algovita®'s features include:

- A user-friendly control design and intuitive operation
- A 24-channel rechargeable IPG that implants in the upper buttock and connects to leads in the epidural space
- A comprehensive lead portfolio that boasts a novel **stretchable coil design and different contact configurations**
- Multiple current sources with the broadest overall parametric range set—pulse width, frequency, and amplitude—of any system currently in the market to enable personalized therapies
- Wireless, portable patient and physician programmers based on the Medical Implant Communication Service (MICS) band that allows external program adjustments

For these reasons, Nuvectra is the worthy recipient of Frost & Sullivan's 2017 North America New

Product Innovation Award in the spinal cord stimulation market.

Each year, Frost & Sullivan presents this award to the company that has developed an innovative element in a product by leveraging leading-edge technologies. The award recognizes the value-added features and benefits of the product and the increased returns on investment it offers customers, which in turn increases customer acquisition and overall market penetration potential.

Frost & Sullivan Best Practices Awards recognize companies in a variety of regional and global markets for demonstrating outstanding achievement and superior performance in areas such as leadership, technological innovation, customer service, and strategic product development.

Industry analysts compare market participants and measure performance through in-depth interviews, analysis, and extensive secondary research to identify best practices in the industry.

Paresthesia-free

One of the terms you hear thrown around when discussing SCS is "Paresthesia Free". What is that? Is it important? I had no clue when I began my research, so here is a little information regarding this.

> *"paresthesia* — electric-shock sensations in the brain that many people call brain zaps.

> *Medical Definition of* **Paresthesia**
> **:** a sensation of pricking, tingling, or creeping on the skin having no objective cause and usually associated with injury or irritation of a sensory nerve or nerve root." (Merriam Webster's dictionary)

"Paresthesia refers to a burning or prickling sensation that is usually felt in the hands, arms, legs, or feet, but can also occur in other parts of the body. The sensation, which happens without warning, is usually painless and described as tingling or numbness, skin crawling, or itching. Most people have experienced temporary paresthesia -- a feeling of "pins and needles" -- at some time in their lives when they have sat with legs crossed for too long, or fallen asleep with an arm crooked under their head. It happens when sustained pressure is placed on a nerve. The feeling quickly goes away once the pressure is relieved. Chronic paresthesia is often a symptom of an underlying neurological disease or traumatic nerve damage. Paresthesia can be caused by disorders affecting the central nervous system, such as stroke and transient ischemic attacks (mini-strokes), multiple sclerosis, transverse myelitis, and encephalitis. A tumor or vascular lesion pressed up against the brain or spinal cord can also cause paresthesia. Nerve entrapment syndromes, such as carpal tunnel syndrome, can damage peripheral nerves and cause paresthesia accompanied by pain. Diagnostic evaluation is based on determining the underlying condition causing the paresthetic sensations." (http://Malacards.org)

"Nuvectra put together a quick comparison chart **on their website** in the investor relations section of their website. It is slide 10 of the March investor presentation. You can look it up, but here is a summary.

- The number of channels ranges from 16 (MDT/STJ) to 32 (BSX). NVTR is in the middle with 24 (either 3 leads of 8 poles or 2 leads of 12 poles). BSX has 36 independent channels. NVTR has 24 independent channels. The others have fewer channels and they aren't independent. Keep in mind that all of the systems have a practical limit to the number of electrodes that can fire simultaneously because there's a limit to how much total amperage can be delivered at the same time. Advantage BSX.

- NVTR has the highest max amplitude at 30mA. MDT is worst at 10.5 mA. Advantage NVTR.

- MDT/STJ is constant voltage. BSX/NVTR is constant current. Constant current is better as tissue impedance changes over time. MDT's next gen will have the option of constant current or constant voltage. I have not tried NVRO. I do not know if it is constant voltage or current. Advantage BSX/NVTR.

- With high frequency you get paresthesia free which is preferable for most patients as they feel nothing as opposed to numb/tingling. MDT/BSX/STJ cap themselves at 1200 Hz. This is probably to avoid getting sued by NVRO who has a patent above 1200 Hz. NVTR has chosen to go up to 2000 MHz. If they were a significant threat, they would probably be sued. Advantage NVRO by a wide margin but again not the same type of device. Within the category, advantage NVTR.

- NVTR has the widest range of pulse width. 20-1500 microseconds. BSX/NVRO are 20-1000 micro seconds. Advantage NVTR.

- The 12 polar extended lead does let you stimulate three dermatomes with the same lead. That is nice.

- Stimulator volume is comparable except for NVRO. The others run between 18 cc (STJ) and 22 cc (BSX). (Cafepharma.com blog post)

X-ray of spine after insertion

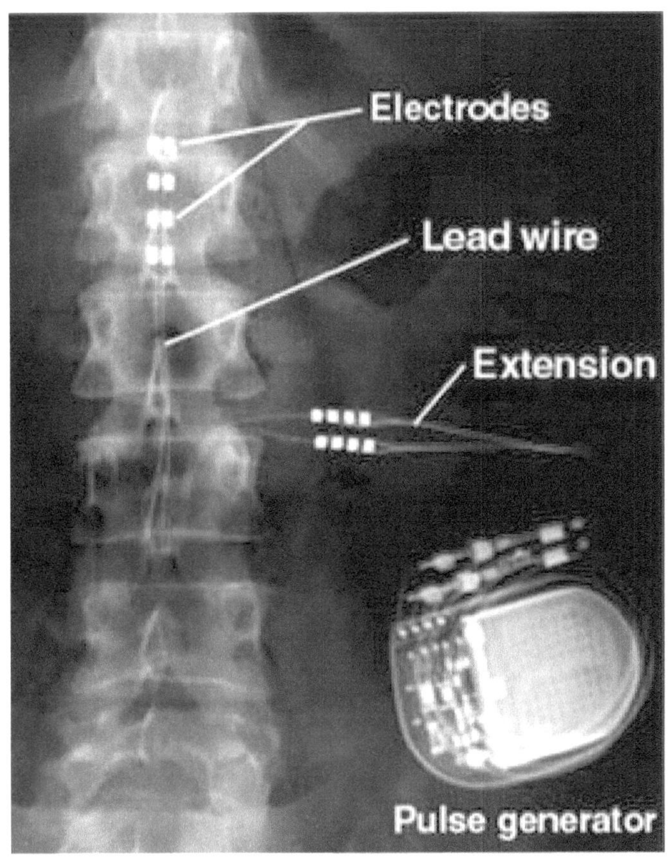

Personal Thoughts:

The above articles were just pieces of the research information I went through, but as you can see it is impressive. This is not to take away from any of the other companies that make these units available. Each seem to do a wonderful job and I realize that you may not have a choice as to what "brand" you have available to you. I have no reason to doubt that each of the major manufactures provide equipment that will take care of your needs, so don't let me put you off on any of them. Again, let me encourage you talk with your health care professional about what units they have available to them and then make an educated decision.

Just as with Boston Scientific, a representative of NuVectra contacted me after I had my consultation with the surgeon. Again the surgeon I chose uses the NuVectra implant.

Again I was impressed at the level of knowledge this representative had and her willingness to answer any questions I might have. She said that she could be contacted pretty much 24/7 via her phone and if she was not available at the time she would get back with me as soon as possible. Since this is the unit I decided upon we have spoken several times on the phone and had some face to face time in the doctor's office.

I want make sure that you to understand that this is a long term commitment. It's not something that you can have removed easily if you change your mind.

The bottom line is that we are talking about a surgical procedure implanting a foreign object into your back and inside of your spinal column. To remove it also would require surgery and unless it is for medical reasons I doubt that your insurance company will pay for the procedure. That's why you need to do some research and think things through before making the commitment for a Spinal Cord Stimulator Implantation.

In doing my research I found that there had been well over a million of these procedures done. But, one of the things I wanted to check on was how people reacted to having the procedure.

I was somewhat surprised that in all of the forums, blogs and general information I ran across I found less than a dozen people who were unhappy with the procedure. I'll write more about this when I share some of my interactions with people who have had the procedure.

That said a lot to me about the success of what was being done. Obviously not everyone who had a complaint would voice it on the Internet, but if you know anything about the Internet you know that people are generally not hesitant to complain if they are unhappy. The secret nature of the Internet somehow makes people feel freer to express their unhappiness.

A COUPLE OF OTHER THINGS YOU MAY WANT TO KNOW…

MRI's and Security Checks

Due to the very nature of having metal and wires inserted into your back you will no longer be able to have MRI's. An MRI uses extremely high magnetic pulses to look through your body's tissue and see the smallest issues you might have. It becomes dangerous to be in the presence of these strong magnetic waves if you have metal in your body.

In a similar way, but not quite so extreme you will want to avoid the metal detectors in airports and other security check areas. The magnet pulses they put out can seriously mess up the delicate computer system/receiver/ transmitter which now reside in your back. The representative told me the results probably would be that the unit shut down.

Yes, they give you a plastic card that will tell everyone you have a Neurostimulation Implant, so yes that will help at the airport, etc.

However I started looking into a medical alert bracelet for that purpose. As I did more research I read of the occasional times where people were incapacitated and taken to the hospital and subjected to an MRI. Does it happen often? No, but I don't want to take a chance. (**Personal note**: The magnetic medical alert bracelets were more attractive to me, but there is a chance that they will interfere with the implant so I chose a stainless steel one).

One of the blog posts I read was from a Firefighter/EMS who said that they almost never look in your wallet for that kind of information. He said it made their job a lot easier and you a lot safer if you had an Alert Bracelet which is easily seen and one of the first things they check.

So, with the idea of rather being safe than sorry I ordered a Medical Alert Bracelet that says, **"NO MRI" "Neurostimulation Implant" "NO Magnet security checks".** Then on the inside I had engraved my doctor's information as well as the customer service number for NuVectra and my unit's ID number as well as an emergency contact number. For me everything was a learning experience. When I began I knew very little about the Spinal Column and how it was put together. Yes, I understood the disk and vertebrae relationship, but not how it all went together.

I found this interesting little chart that fills in a couple of the blanks as far as how the spine is described.

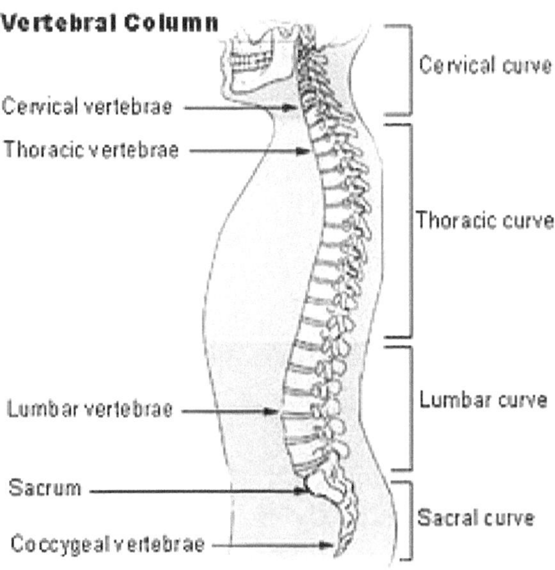

The Surgery

I can't say that I was particularly worried about having the surgery; however this was my first surgery and was unprepared to some degree as to how it would affect me.

Preparing for the surgery

In all honesty, the surgery part went off without a hitch. It was the standard pre-op with no eating or drinking after midnight, etc.

We arrived early and they took my vitals, hooked up an IV port, treated my nose for MERSA, (just in case) they said it was easily spread and always took this precaution.

A Side thought on my pain:

During the question and answer part of getting me ready they ask several questions dutifully writing my answers down on their clipboard/chart. One of the questions they ask was about my pain level that morning. I remember telling them, (on a scale of 1-10 with 10 being the highest), that the pain level was about 7-8.

I hadn't remembered that incident until 3 weeks later when I had the staples removed. The nurse asked more questions for my chart and one of them again was about my pain level. I hadn't thought about it that day and was actually surprised when she asked me the question. My response was that I was at a level 1, maybe a 2… In other words, I wasn't even thinking about it. How quickly I had become used to being more pain free…. Does that mean I never have pain? NO, but it is reduced and mostly controllable.

Back to the surgery…

When the time came, they wheeled me down the hall in to the operation room, placed a mask over my face and told me to breath. That was the last thing I remembered until I woke up in recovery.

The Procedure:

One of the things I did not expect and did not think to ask, (again this was my first surgery), was about the actual procedure itself.

Because of my interaction with other folks who had the procedure I just assumed mine would be the same, one incision and some stitches.

What actually happened was that there were two incisions and lots of staples, (in the most inconvenient places when sitting).

The doctor made one vertical incision about 3 inches long at the base of my spine and another horizontal incision about 3 inches long over my right kidney. The vertical incision was to insert the wires into my spinal column and the horizontal incision was to insert the control unit and then fished the wires over between the two and stapled me shut. There were 9 staples in each incision.

After Surgery and the Recovery:

The surgery was considered "*Out Patient*," which means the whole procedure from the time of check in to discharge took about 6 hours. They of course keep you in recovery until you are somewhat coherent. My wife (and driver), said that she helped me dress and that I talked to her after and on the way home, but I honestly have no memory of the trip or even arriving home. So, I was ***feeling no pain*** and slept the rest of the afternoon and evening.

The post operative instructions were to rest and leave the dressing on for 3 days then we could change them. No stretching, no bending, no lifting over 5 pounds and no driving until released by the doctor. I personally was surprised at that time to learn about the 2 incisions I had and all of the staples, but not upset. It's just part of the procedure to get me feeling better; I just had not expected them.

The Results: immediate, long term

When they implant the Spinal Cord Stimulator they do a basic programming of the unit. You have a remote control which allows you some control over the unit and intensity of the stimulation. At the time of the surgery they also made an appointment to go meet with the NuVectra representative/technician

after a week to do some further programming for the
Spinal Cord Stimulator. That went well and they
gave me a second preset program which addressed
some specific areas of weakness and pain.

To be honest in the beginning the pain from the
surgery itself was a big distraction from the actual
functioning of the stimulator. It took about 3 days for
the pain to reduce enough to be able to actually tell a
difference with the stimulator.

When my wife began changing my dressings we
could see more of what the doctor did and how it
affected me. (*My wife took pictures with my phone
camera so that I could see what was going on shown
later*).

There was just the normal small amount of bleeding
at both incisions, but at the one incision over my
right kidney the soreness continued for a couple of
weeks. In fact I developed a large bruise over that
area. They open the skin there and insert the control
unit, roughly 2 inches by 2.5 inches and about 3/16
inch thick. I was not concerned or surprised about the
bruising once I thought about it, it made sense.

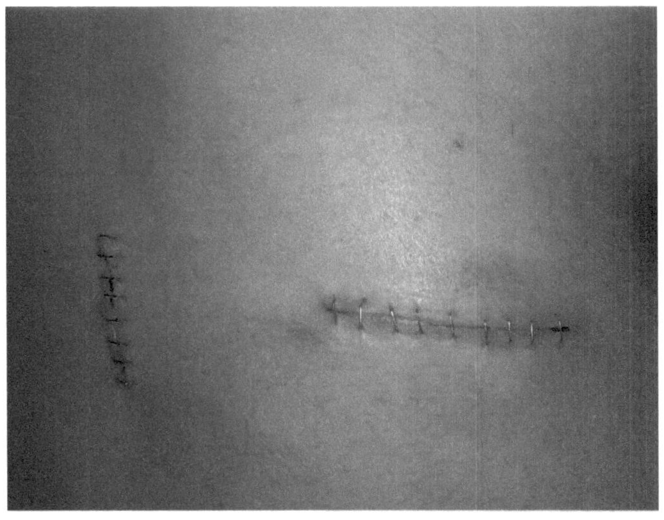

After 3 weeks the bruising pretty much faded, but it was still sensitive to the touch with just a light bit of blood leaking in one area. My wife, (who is usually right), said it's because I refused to "be good" and did many of the things they told me not to such as bending and stretching. I guess that was because my pain level was less and I began feeling like doing things for the first time in over a year.

After 3 weeks the staples came out and I was so glad for that. The staples were in the exact position where you lean when you sit on almost anything. Using a pillow to prop up your upper back so as not to place pressure on your lower back helped. We also discovered that an office chair with the upper back support, but no lower back in the chair worked well. It continued to remain very tender where the control unit is placed for a while longer.

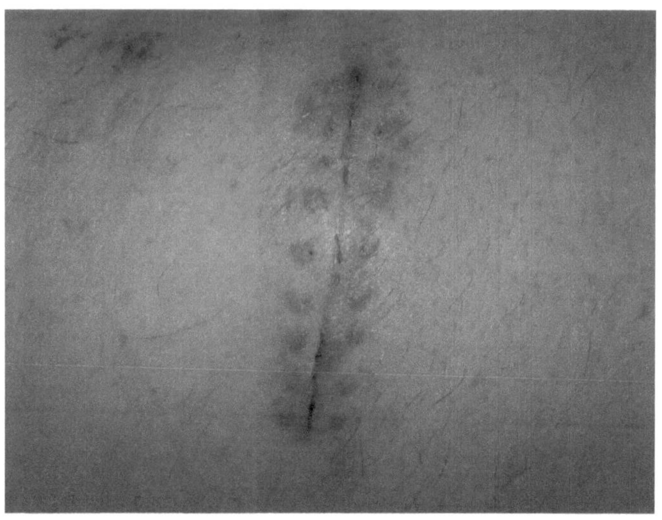

By week 5 the areas on my back were completely
healed, but the area over my right kidney where the
actual control unit is at was still tender from time to
time. Sitting on hard surfaces were still a problem
and I carried a small pillow with me to help with that
problem.

What can you expect?

That is truly a question that can't be answered. Each and every person is different. I wish that someone could tell us or promise us exactly what would happen, but the truth is that they can't. I can share what has happened with me so far and with a few others. Maybe that can give you some hope, because that is what this procedure is all about isn't it? It's about hope that we can be at least more pain free than we are at the present. For me it has worked and hopefully it will for you also.

For example, this morning I woke up with pretty much no pain, but that is how it is when I'm in bed. After a few minutes of being up and moving around I started having sharp stabbing pains in my lower back. What did I do? I turned my Stimulator up with my handy remote control and it dialed back my pain. Did it completely remove it? No! But it went from sharp stabbing to a light ache, kind of like an over used muscle.

I showered and got ready for church and drove there, interacted with many of my fellow worshipers with almost no pain. It did not debilitate me, in fact much of the time I did not even notice it.

However three days ago I did something I shouldn't have and my back hurt all day. It was not at the same level as it would have been without the stimulator, but there was a pain there that said, "Sit down and take it easy today/" To which I said, "Good idea," and did.

For me the experience has been a good one and worth the experience of having the surgery to implant it.

So far what has changed for me?

1. Greatly reduced back pain, from a level 8 to a level 2 most of the time.

2. Numbness in my toes and feet is gone.

3. The weakness in my right leg which caused me to stumble is almost completely gone. I have a small limp on occasion, but I no longer use a cane and feel that I am getting stronger as each day goes by.

4. I am able to once again do some of the things I was forced to give up like household chores, maintenance, etc. I hope to be able to mow my own yard next spring and work in my flower

beds. I also help a lot with the cooking, (which I enjoy doing and my wife says she enjoys not doing after 52 years of marriage.)

5. I am able go to the YMCA and walk and use some of the equipment such as the stationary bike and treadmill.

6. I was unable to raise my right foot high enough to put on my sock. For the most part now I can put on my own sock, though I still can't raise my leg as high as I used to be able. And I can put my socks on by myself.

7. My balance has improved quite a bit. Rather than having to lean on things while dressing or showering I can stand on my own now.

I really didn't understand the description of the vertebra before it involved me personally. Here is how it is laid out.

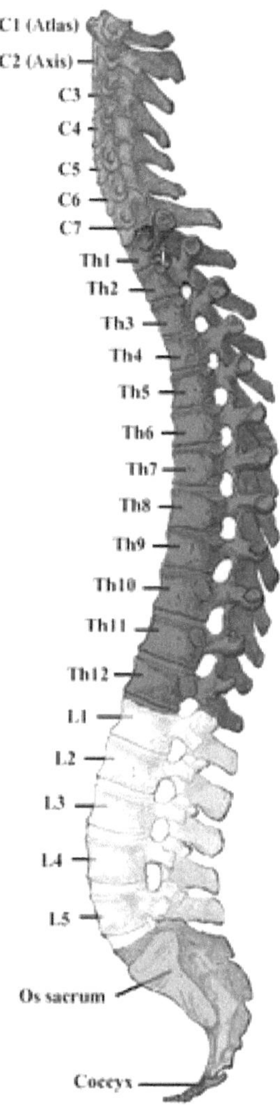

SOME CONTINUING PROBLEMS AND CONSIDERATIONS

One of the things the doctor cautioned me about is that the Spinal Cord Stimulator will not "fix" my damaged spine; it only helps me deal with the pain. So I will never be able to go back to a job such as the lumber/appliance store.

1. I have a lifting weight limit of around 10 pounds, (though I occasionally lift a little more I am ever vigilant. I don't want to injure myself further.)

2. I have trouble sitting for long periods of time on hard surfaces such as church pews or folding chairs. I carry a light pillow with me on those occasions, but still after awhile the pain comes. At home an office chair works well with the lower back open.

3. I remember during my research asking those who already had a simulator, "How do you know if you reinjure yourself if the stimulator masks the pain?" The response was, "You will know!" They were right, if you over do it your back pain will let you know. It does not remove all pain, it helps control the pain. Today I went outside and spread fertilizer on

the yard. I felt pretty good when I started. After I came in and showered I had to sit and recoup for awhile and turn the stimulator up a little. After a couple of hours resting I was alright.

4. It will take awhile for you to learn to live with your Spinal Cord Stimulator unit. The remote control is really simple and shouldn't give you any trouble learning how to read it and adjust the settings.

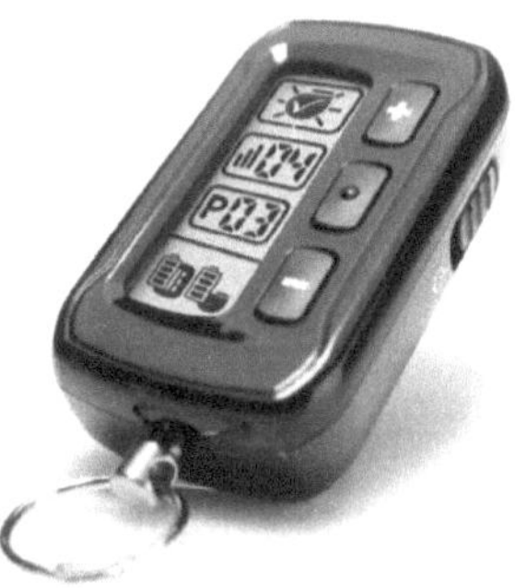

Example of remote control unit

5. I am still getting comfortable with my SCS unit and how best to adjust it.

6. Because of my weakness in my right leg I have more problems with it if I have been on my feet for a long time or am walking or

shopping for extended periods of time. I still
have to think about it and remember to change
my program to the one that focuses on my
right leg and lower back in that area. I think
that it will become more a "second nature" as
they say as time goes on. At night when I go to
bed I turn the stimulation down as I have less
pain while lying in bed.

7. Learning to position your charger is a
   challenge at first, but after a few tries you will
   get the hang of it.

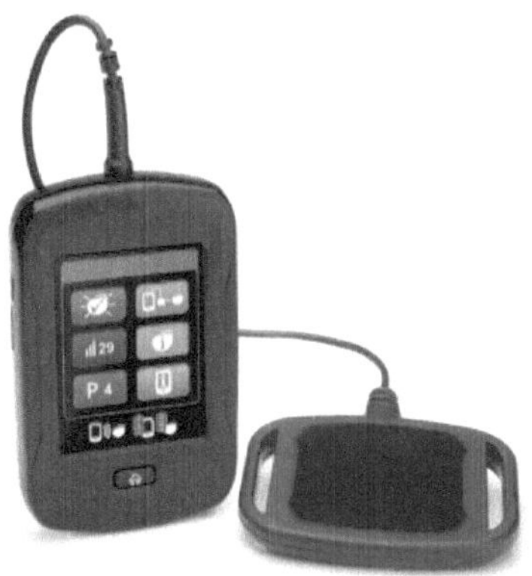

Example of charging unit

8. I have learned that sitting on a hard seat for an
   extended period of time still brings me pain.
   Pews, hard chairs and things like that. By a
   long period of time I mean 45 minutes to an
   hour.

SPECIAL CHALLENGES FOR THOSE WITH MORE SERIOUS SPINE ISSUES.

I have talked with some who have had previous procedures on their backs/spines. Things like areas being fused or cages to rebuild the spine.

One of our church friends, Judy, has this situation. She had had 10 surgeries and desperately waned to try the Spinal Cord Stimulator.

She has had numerous procedures to her spine: plates and screws, disks replaced, bone bridges as well as dealing with lots of arthritics which makes it difficult to get the wires in the spine.

She had to try and find a specialist that would attempt this procedure for her. She has had all of the required steps and finally had the surgery.

Her comment was this: "Before I went into surgery my pain level was 10+, immediately after my surgery my pain level was 0-1." Wow, what wonderful results for this lovely lady who has been in pain for so long.

She did have one complication with her surgery. Because of the condition of her spine they had to manipulate her body to get the wires where they needed to go. This meant they had to lift and twist her body to get the wires through some of the previous surgery areas. In doing this they pulled a muscle or injured a nerve in her side. She is on medication for that, but the doctors assure her it should clear up. She said it is the best thing she ever did.

Don't give up if you think, (or your doctor thinks), the stimulator might help you. You may have to do some research or perhaps your current doctor can help you to find a surgeon who will do the procedure for you. Again, it is your body and you have to take responsibility for it.

What others have to say who have had the SCS Implanted.

Rather than rely completely on second hand information, blogs, forums, etc. I wanted to get some face to face time with people who actually had a stimulator implanted. I was pleased that everyone I spoke with basically said it was the best decision they had made and were quite happy with their stimulator no matter what brand it was. Following is not a complete list of everyone I spoke with, but it is a sampling.

Betty had a degenerative condition and could hardly walk from the pain. She was unable to raise her legs to step up at a curb and kind of shuffled when she walked. She was in constant pain. Much of the time she was confined to her home. She has had the SCS implant for a little over a year and says it is wonderful! She can walk and get out of the house whenever she wishes now. The only problem she has had was one time when she forgot to charge the unit. It took her awhile to figure out why it wasn't working, but other than that she loves it.

Becky injured her back at work, (in a steel foundry). She was in pretty much constant pain. She has had her SCS implant for a couple of years now and also says it was one of the best decisions she ever made. She has complete mobility. She was very encouraging to me, urging me to consider the procedure when I talked with her.

Charles has a less favorable report. He has had his implant for a couple of years and though he says it helps, he still has pain. He is around 70 years old and is very active. He does his own yard work, washes his car does his own home maintenance and pretty much anything he wants. He also goes to the YMCA several times a week and works out. He recommends the pool for water therapy. As he expressed it to me he is not as happy with his unit as he had hoped, but he also was the first one that encouraged me to look into it more seriously.

<u>Debby</u> has had her unit for several years and loves it. She also had a back injury and says that she couldn't function without her SCS implant. Before she got it she was pretty much house bound.

<u>Bob</u> is one of those exceptions we rarely hear about. I had known Bob for about 30 years. He had his implant about 10 years ago and was unhappy with it from the start. He was a retired over the road truck driver. He spent many long hours driving his truck across the country which eventually caused damage to his spine. It seems he did not get the relief he had expected and really didn't like the idea of having the wires in his spine and the control unit in his back. Bob eventually had his SCS unit removed.

Epilog

At this point when someone asks how I am doing my reply is generally, "***Just Great***!" My wife made the comment, "***It is sure good to have my husband back again***." I asked her what she meant and she said, "***You are laughing, kidding, and smiling once again***."

I hadn't thought about it or the changes this has made in my life already. Someone asked me at church yesterday how I was doing and I said, "Just Great!" and then did a little jig to show them. I always liked to kid around with people, but hadn't done that for awhile and hadn't even noticed it myself.

Several people have told me, I know you are doing better I can see it in your face. My brother who lives out of state told me: "***I know you are doing better, I can hear it in your voice***."

Will you have the same level of success? I have no idea, but for me it has made a huge difference.

Web Forums/Resources

Below you will find only a few of the many resources available if you search the Internet. Perhaps this will make your research a little easier.

1. WebMD - https://forums.webmd.com/3/pain-management-exchange/forum/2961

2. Pain Clinic Advisor - https://www.clinicalpainadvisor.com/interventional-pain-management/high-vs-low-frequency-spinal-cord-stimulation-for-the-long-term-treatment-of-back-and-leg-pain/article/523871/

3. YouTube video of Spinal Cord Stimulator Surgery (Note this is graphic and shows you everything). –

4. Spine Health Forum - https://www.spine-health.com/seek?query=spinal+cord+stimulator

5. Café Pharma Forum - http://www.cafepharma.com/boards/search/7228296/?q=spinal+cord+stimulator&o=date&c%5bnode%5d=231

Something extra from my blog:

ME, Version 2.0, Cyborg adaptation…

Well, at my age I've done and experienced a lot of things. Living life is really about change and adjustment to times, events and places. For the past 12 months I have gone from a healthy active life to being permanently disabled. As I said, I've experienced a lot, but even so I find that there is always something new right around the corner. For example, this week I had my first surgery in a hospital and became a Cyborg.

If it weren't for the pain experienced with the actual surgery, I would think it is a really neat thing. (Third day now and the pain is better). After all, I've been a lifelong fan of Science Fiction stories, but never thought I would actually join the Cyborg crowd. Now, if you are wondering, a Cyborg is defined the following way: "***A person whose physiological function is aided by or dependent upon a mechanical or electronic device***". Since I now have a small computer implanted in my back and electronic leads in my spine I guess I qualify (smile).

It's amazing the way that technology can change your life, sometimes for the better, sometimes not. But as much as this new piece of technology is helping me already, it's not the help I'm looking for. I'm looking for something more permanent. I'm looking for, (longing for as some would say), that time when this physical body will no longer matter.

1 Corinthians 15:51-53 encourages us with these words:
"we shall all be changed,
In a moment, in the twinkling of an eye, at the last trump:
for the trumpet shall sound, and the dead shall be raised

incorruptible, and we shall be changed. For this corruptible must put on incorruption, and this mortal must put on immortality."

Thinking about these verses the words, "***Changed***," "***Incorruptible***," "***Immortality***", stand out to me. Those are important words in the life of a Christian aren't they? You see they told me that my new Cyborg computer battery has an expected life span of 5-10 years and it has to be recharged every few days. None of those words from 1 Corinthians apply to what I now have or am and I want something better, more permanent. Don't you?

That's what is so great is something else I have implanted in me; it's the Holy Spirit and Jesus living in me that confirms the promise to me that I will be "changed, incorruptible and immortal". There is an old song I love that proclaims, "I'm going to live forever, I'm going to die no never, Jesus died on the cross for me and I'm going to live forever". How are you doing in that relationship to the one who offers you life eternal? Cybernetic implants are great, but Jesus is better!

Russ Lawson

Blog: http://myunexpectedadventure.com

Blog: http://healthhopeandherbs.com

A request for you

As you can see, gathering all of the information into one place took a lot of effort. As an independent author on Amazon I really make very little profit from the sale of each book so I could use all of the help I can get.

My request is this, if you have found this book to be informative or helpful, please go to the order page on Amazon and add a review of this book. It is important to how the book is ranked by Amazon and perhaps even whether I receive revenue from the sale of the book.

Go to Amazon.com Kindle books and search for Russ Lawson and it will take you to the page with my books. You can click on the book and then leave a review at the bottom.

Or go here:

https://www.amazon.com/s/ref=nb_sb_noss?url=search-alias%3Ddigital-text&field-keywords=russ+lawson

It doesn't have to be a long review at all, but it truly would be appreciated.

Thank you for taking the time to read this book of mine.

Russ Lawson